Cape Fear

TABLE OF CONTENTS

1. Messy/Sucio
2. Perseverance/Perseverancia
3. Believe/Creer
4. Choice/Eleccion
5. Door/Puerta
6. Change/Cambio
7. World / El Mundo
8. Positive Affirmations/Afirmaciones positivas
9. Fall Seven, Rise Eight/ Caer siete, subir ocho
10. Hand-Pick/Escogido a mano
11. Struggle/Lucha
12. Travelers/Viajero
13. Nothing/Nada
14. Intention Intencion
15. Playful/Jugueton
16. Artistry/El Arte
17. River and Sea/ Rio y Mar
18. Sentiment/Sentimiento
19. Cape Fear/Rio del Cabo Mieda
20. Whole/ Completo
21. Spirit/Espiritu
22. Complete/Completo
23. Time/Hora
24. Peaceful/Pacific
25. Create It/Crearlo
26. Cling/Afferan
27. Free/Libre
28. Trust/Confia
29. Dream/Sueno
30. Eden/Eden
31. Survival/La Supervivencia
32. Cost/Costo

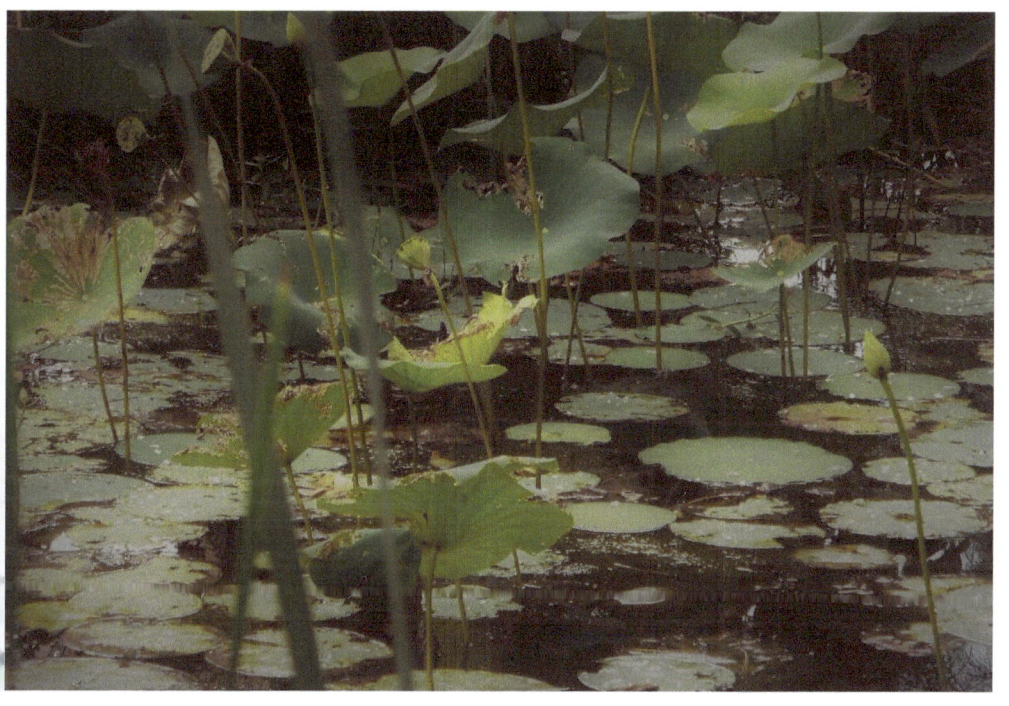

Messy

Public Appearance

Urbane

Worldly

Meditative

State

Serenity

With

The

Messy

Of

My

Life

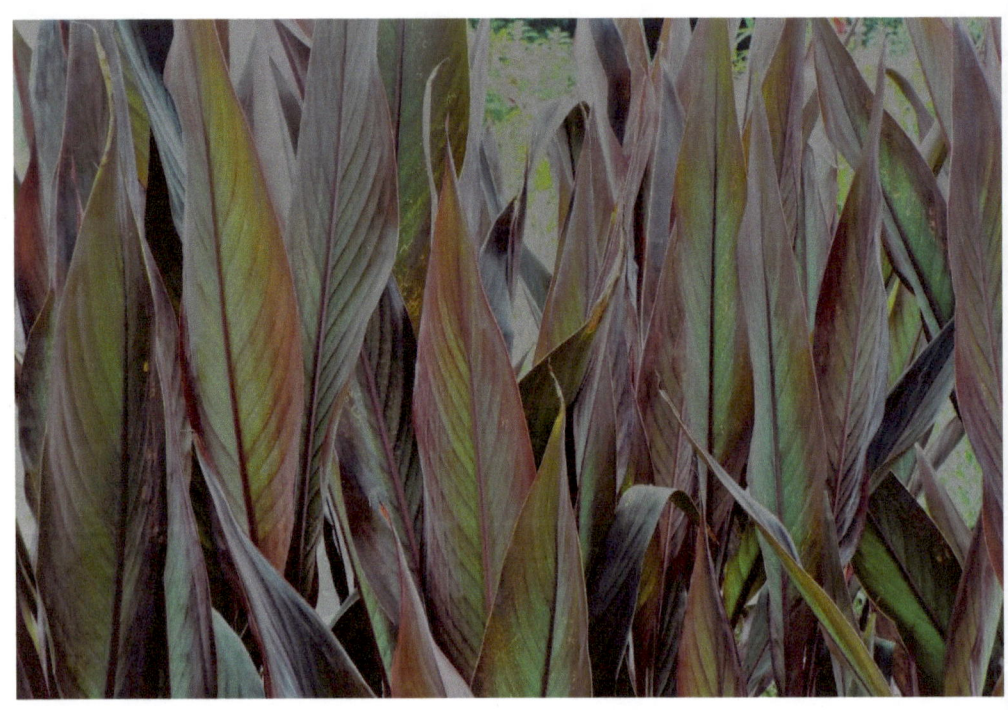

A great accomplishment takes a lot of perseverance

Un gran logro reqiere mucha perseverancia

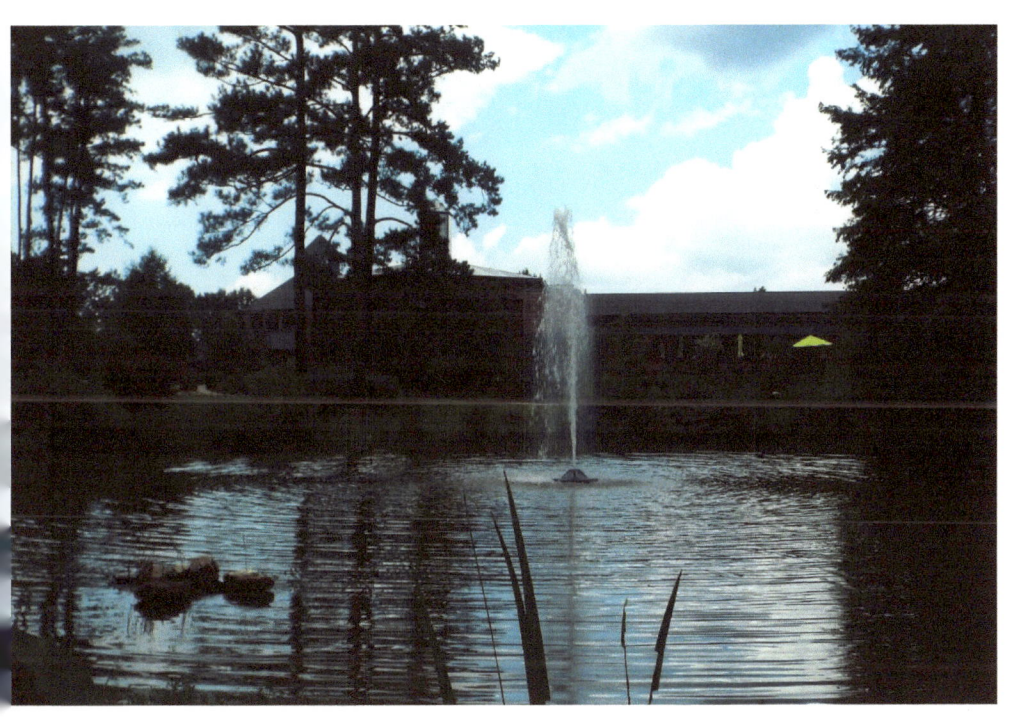

Believe that you are becoming the best you can be

Cree en que te estas conviertiendo en la major version de tu persona

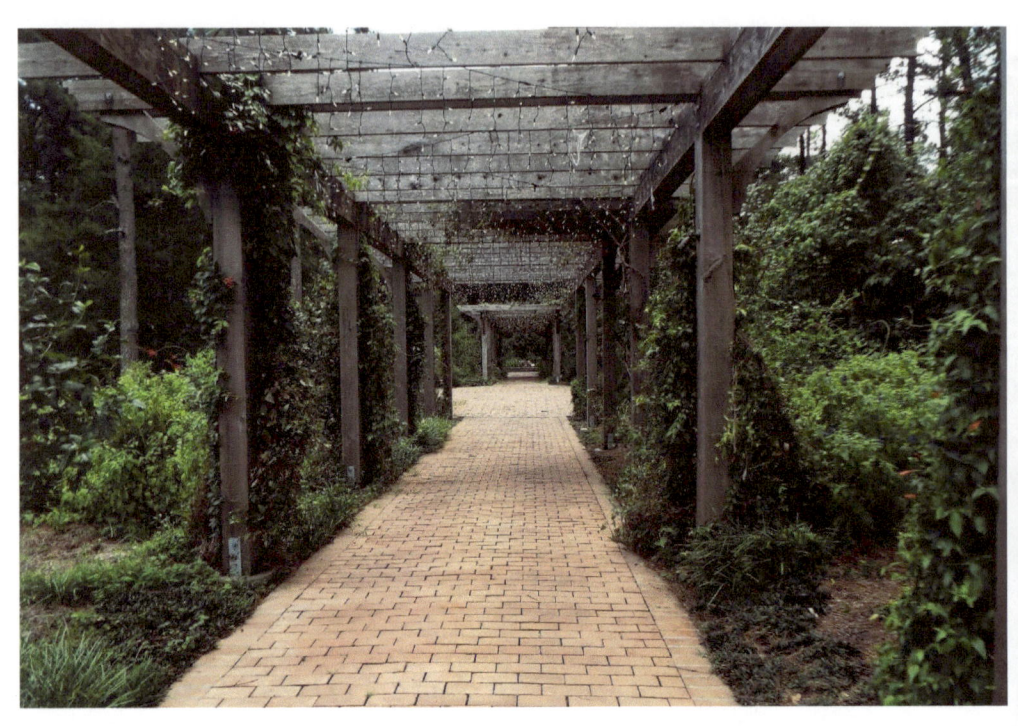

We all have a choice

Todos temenos las opcion

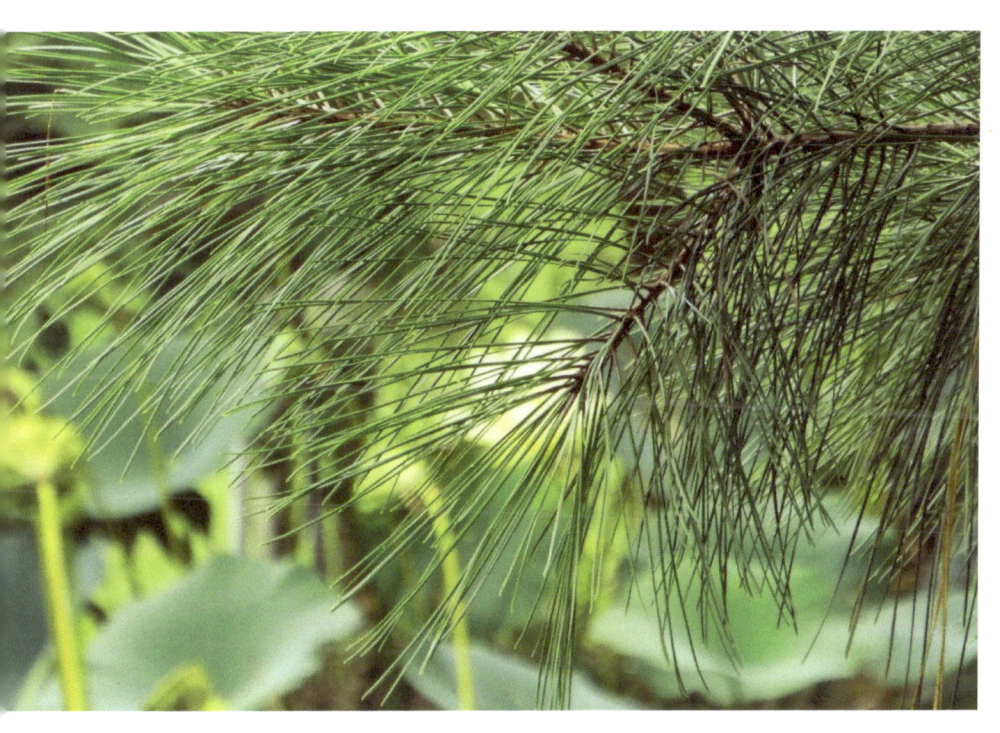

When God closes a door, God opens a window

Cuando Dios Cierra una Puerta, siempre abre una ventana

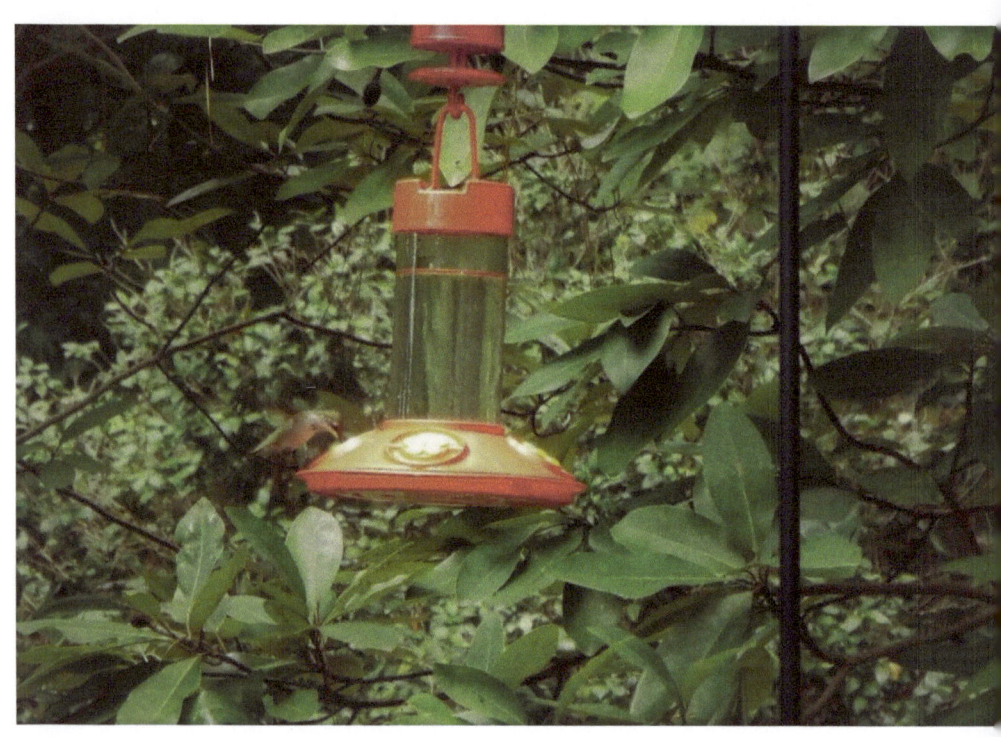

Be the change you wish to see in the world

Se el cambio que deseas ver en el mundo

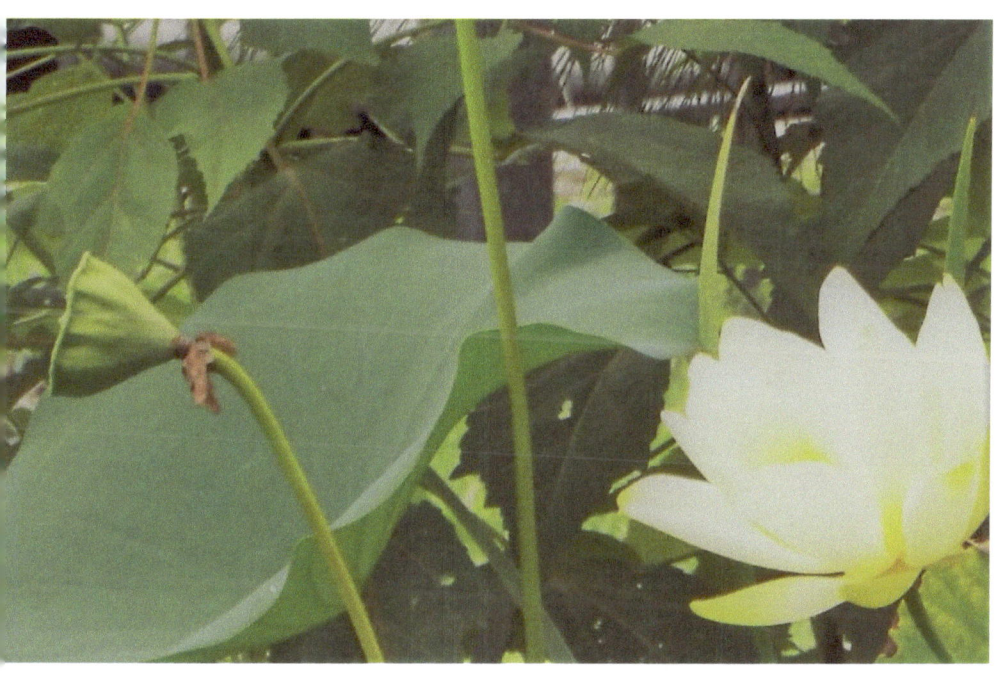

Give the world the best you have, and the best will come back to you

Dale al mundo lo major que tienes y lo major volvera a ti

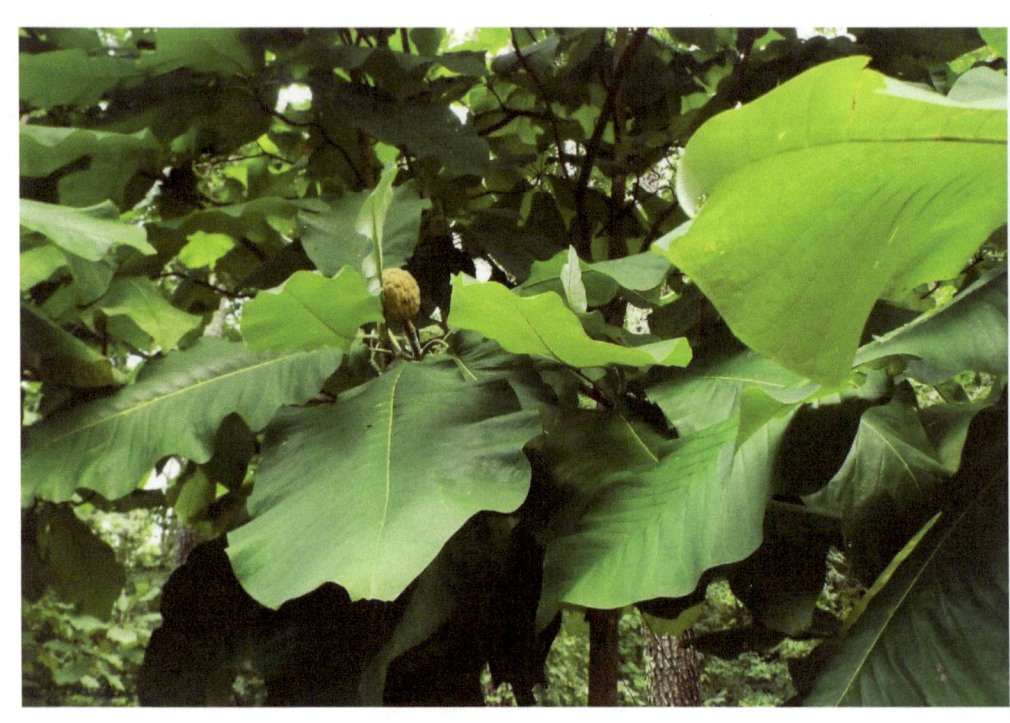

Make a positive affirmation a way of life

Haz que tus afirmaciones postivas sean un estilo de vida

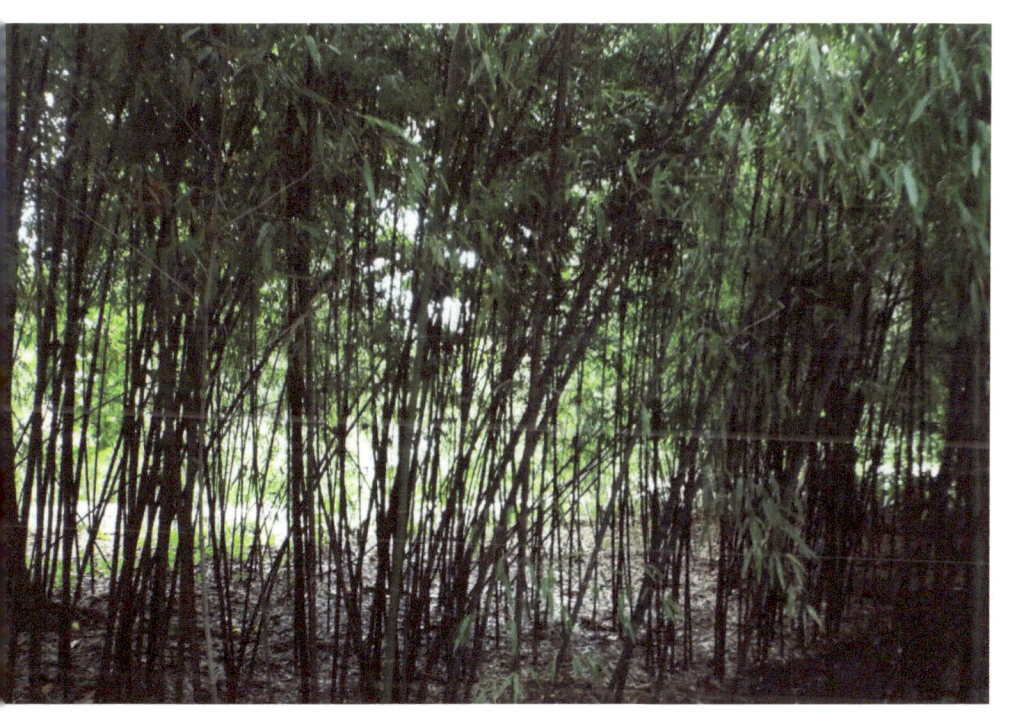

Successful people believe that failure is an unexpected outcome.

Las personas exitosas creen que el fracas es en resulatado inesperado.

Fall seven, Rise eight

Caer siete, subir ocho

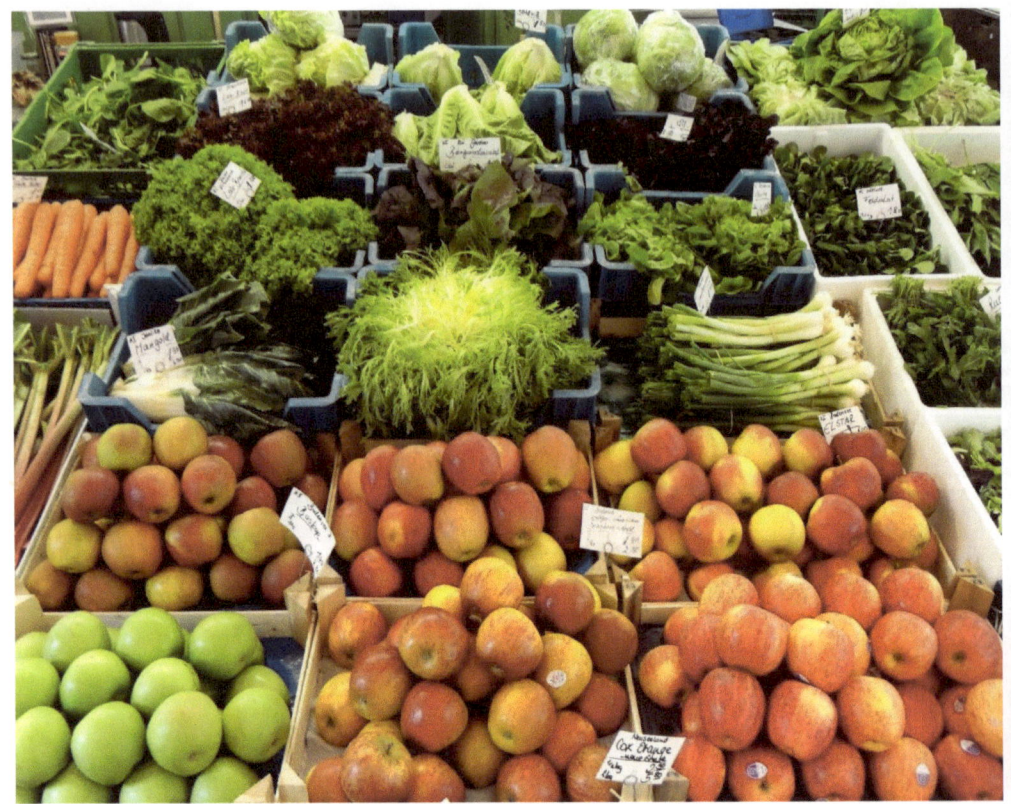

[This Photo](#) by Unknown Author is licensed under [CC BY-SA](#)

Hand-Picked

How many of us have asked the question about how the produce reaches the stores? We see photos of farmers and produce staff in the store, our awareness stops at the photos. Most of the produce within the store is hand-picked on a farm or nursery. 85% of our fruits and vegetables are harvested by hand.

One can not use a machine to pick strawberries, apples, peaches, sweet potatoes, corn, bell peppers, peppers, carrots, onions, peanuts, collard greens, Christmas trees, or salad. A machine can not plant and nurture the plants to mature growth. A machine can not nurture hogs or chickens.

Many people believe migrant workers only work and live in California. California is just one location. Migrant workers are mobile people that move with the agricultural season. They reside in temporary housing while working the fields. North Carolina is sixth in the United States for a significant number of migrant workers. Farmworkers have decreased in North Carolina during the past twenty years, however migrant workers have doubled in the past twenty years. 94% of migrant workers are native Spanish speaking males. The migrant workers have replaced sharecroppers, African slaves, tenant farmers, and indentured servants. The migrant workers are the backbone of the agricultural industry of North Carolina since the 1900's.

The families of these men are in their home country. The men can work under the status of "guest worker" in the H2A. The program provides a temporary work visa designed specifically for agricultural workers in the United States. The seasonal farmworkers reside in the community. Popular opinion may be correct about the legal status of some of the migrant workers, according to the Department of Labor reports that 53% of farmworkers nationally are undocumented (working without legal authorization) 25% are American citizens and 21% are permanent residents. The migrant worker and seasonal farmworkers are usually hired by crew leaders. The crew leaders are the intermediaries between the growers and workers. (Facts About North Carolina Farmworkers-Student Action with Farmworkers>content)

The wages of the migrant and seasonal farmworker range from 10,000 to 5,000 per year. The federal poverty line is 10,830 per individual and 22.050 for a family of four. Low wages/NFWM/National Farm Ministry-fwn.org>resources>low wages)

Seasonal farmworkers reside in the community. Jacqueline Castillo, 19 stated, she was picking cotton at the age of seven in Wayne County, (55 miles from Raleigh, North Carolina). Jacqueline, her mother and siblings would awaken at 4:30, take the van to the field and pick tobacco. Jacqueline has developed the disease called "The Green Monster." The Green Monster is the absorption of nicotine through the skin. She also has a permanently dislocated left arm. The laws say, yes, a child can pick tobacco, Jacqueline Castillo, a worker says, yes. Children are among the most of NC's immigrant farm workers-The New &

Observer>article160293514-https://www.newaobserver.com. "If their parent is employed on a farm or gives them permission, kids under 12 can work in non-hazardous jobs on farms exempt from Fair Labor Standards Act of minimum wage. "(Ibid) Nicotine poisoning is non-hazardous?

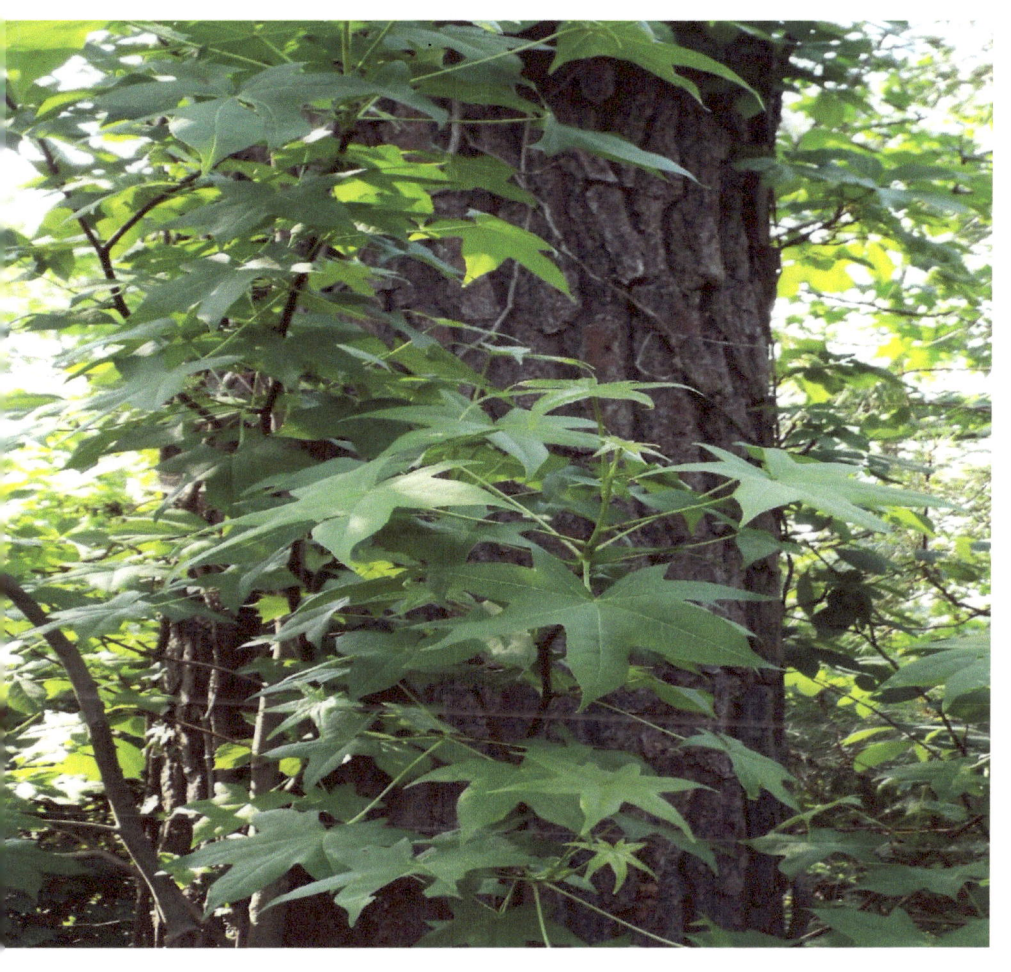

Struggle

In 1966, Martin Luther King was expanding the Civil Rights movement to the "Deep North" in Chicago, Illinois. He chose to reside in a poverty area of the city with the poverty area challenges such as roaches. Fair housing was one of the issues for the urban face of the Civil Rights movement. Cesar Chavez was challenging pesticide poisoning and maltreatment of the Filipino and Mexican farm workers in Delano, California. March 1966, the Filipino and California (capital of California) to create national attention to the migrant worker issues.

brothers in the fight for equality, I extend a hand of fellowship and good will and wish continuing success to you and your members. The fight for equality must be fought on many fronts-in the urban slums, in the sweat shops of the factories and fields. Our separate struggles are really one- struggle for freedom, for dignity, and for humanity. You and your fellow workers have demonstrated your commitment to righting grievous wrongs placed upon exploited people. We are together with you in spirit and in determination that our dreams for a better tomorrow will be realized." (Read the 1966 Telegram MLK Sent Cesar Chavez-Remezcla>culture>1966>mlk-cesar-chavez)

Cesar Chavez and the emerging United Farm Workers Union was not an overnight success with addressing the economic and social equality issues. Cesar Chavez began 25-day fast for non-violence during February -March 1968. Chavez and the emerging United Farm Workers Union garnered support from Andy Young, Jesse Jackson, Coretta Scott King, and Ralph Abernathy. The Chavez and King never met face to face, however the 1968 telegram from King communicated respect, "I am deeply moved by your courage in fasting as your personal sacrifice for justice through non-violence. Your past and present commitment is eloquent testimony to the impotence of violent reprisal. You stand today as a living example of the Ghandian tradition with its great force for social progress and its healing spiritual powers. My colleagues and I commend you for your bravery, salute you for your indefatigable work against poverty and injustice, and pray for your health and your continuing service as one of the outstanding men of America. The plight of your people and ours is so grave that we all desperately need the inspiring example and effective leadership you have given." (Dr. King's telegram to Cesar Chavez during his 1968 fast…. https://ufw.org)

 In 1962, Delores Huerta, co-founder of the United Farm Workers was a tough negotiator and skilled organizer. Cesar Chavez was a dynamic leader and speaker. They were a formidable team. The team work of Chavez and Huerta gave the migrant workers the right to negotiate with the growers. The right entailed 31 years of struggle.

The current trend for migrant workers and growers is crew leaders. The Crew leaders are the middle persons between the migrant workers and the growers

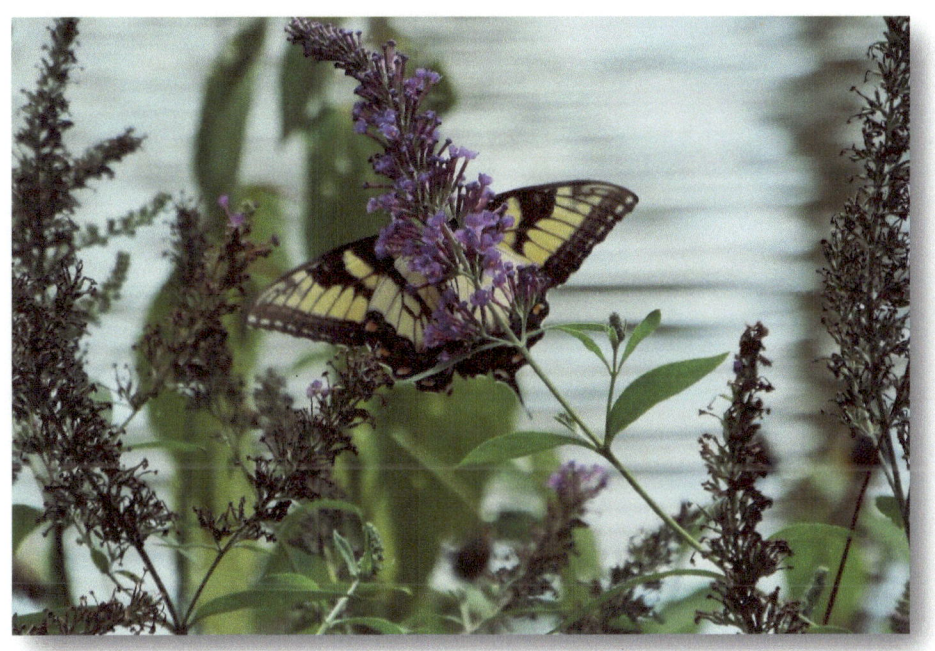

Travelers, it is late. Life's sun is going to set. During the brief days that you have strength, be quick and spare no efforts of your wings.

Rumi

Viajeros, es tarde, el sol de la vida se va a poner, durante los breves dias que tienes fuerza, ser rapido, no escatimes esfuerzos de tus alas

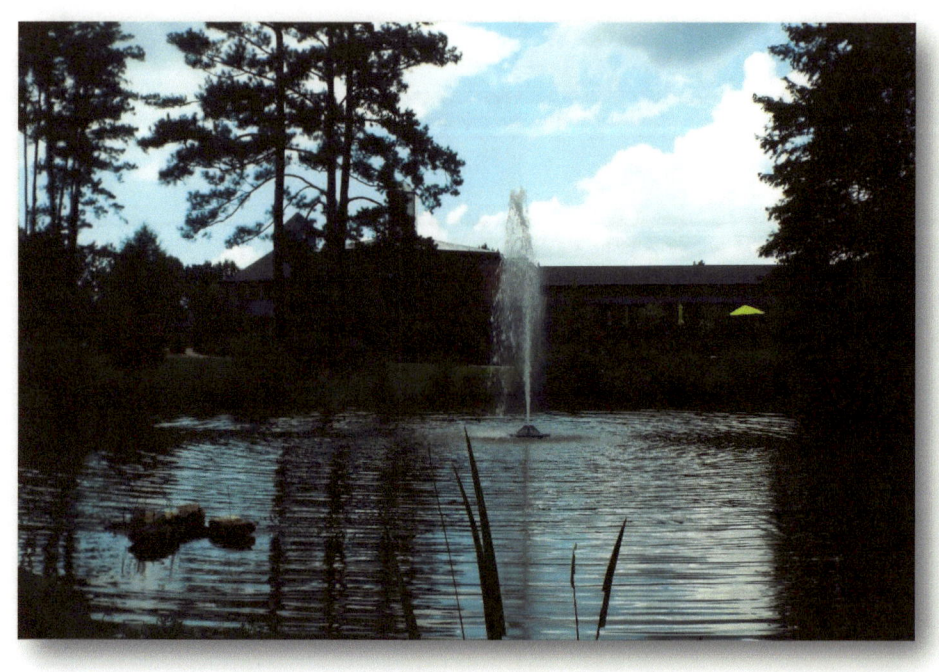

We come from nothing, scattering stars like dust

Venimos de la nada, esparciendo estrellas como el polvo

                                        Rumi

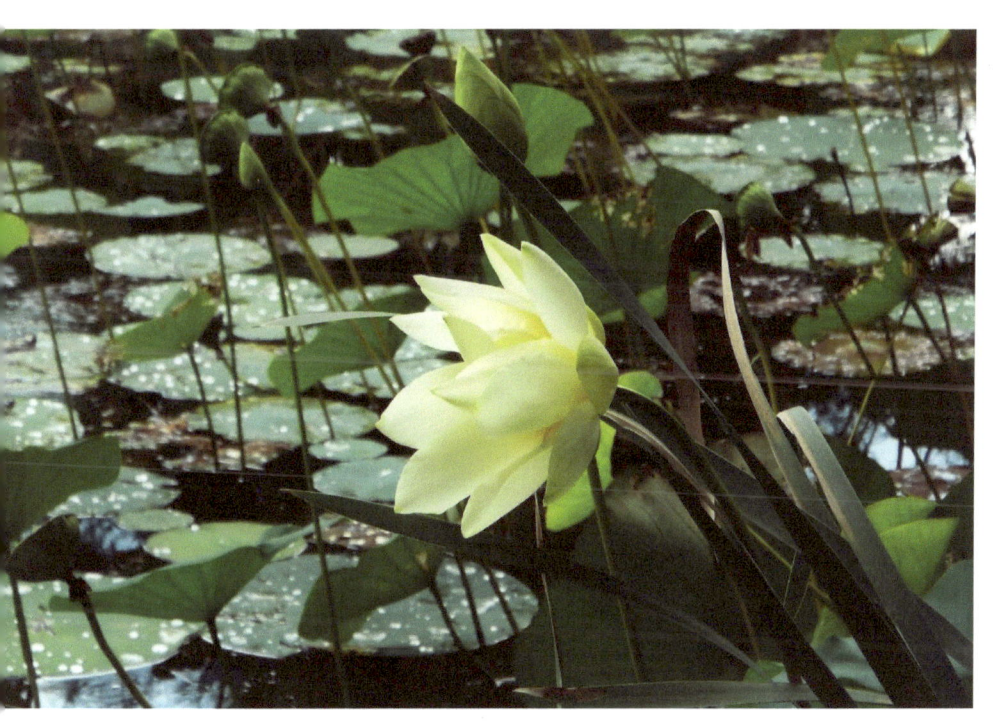

tention align and design with the Source

tencion alinear y disenar con La Fuente

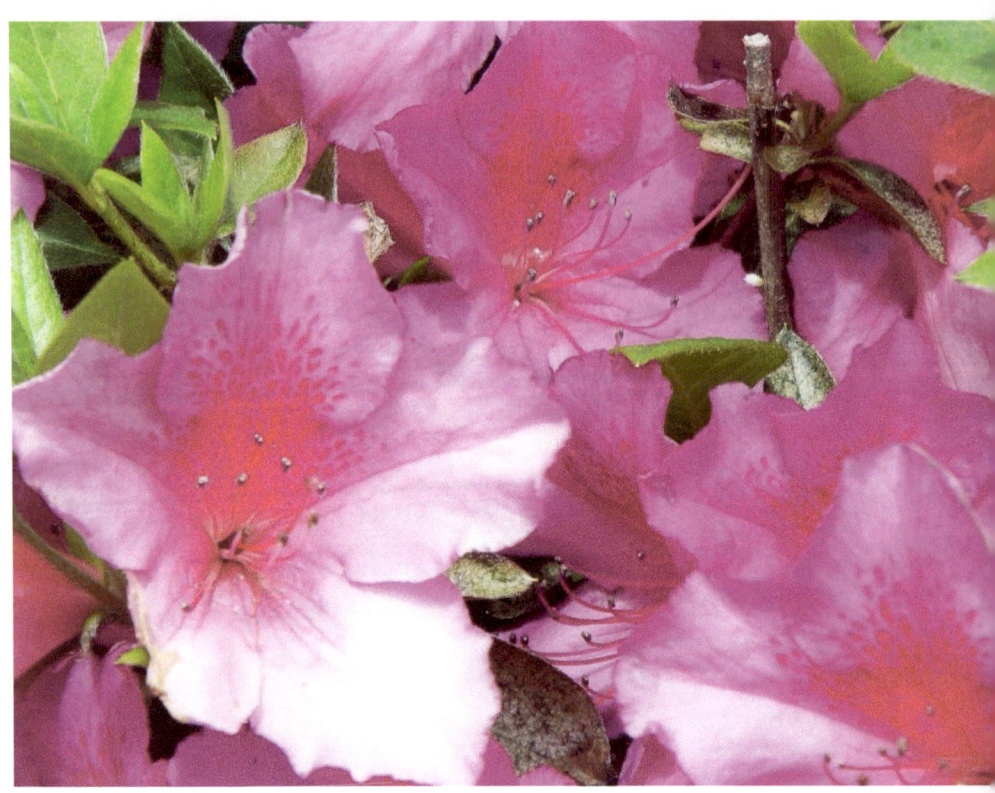

Pretty, pink

Playful

In the summer

Sun

Bonita, rosa

Jugueton

En el sol

De Verano

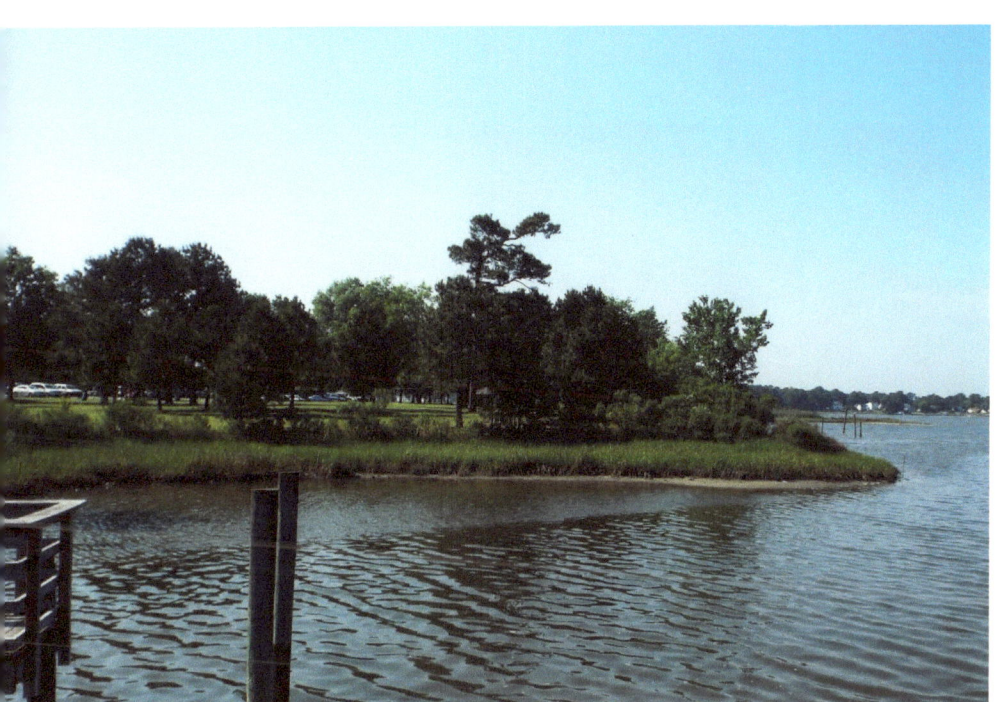

Bennett's Creek

Sand crabs/Cangrejos de arenas

Ebb/ Marea alta y baja

High

Tides

Flowing/Flyendo hacia

To

James River/El rio James

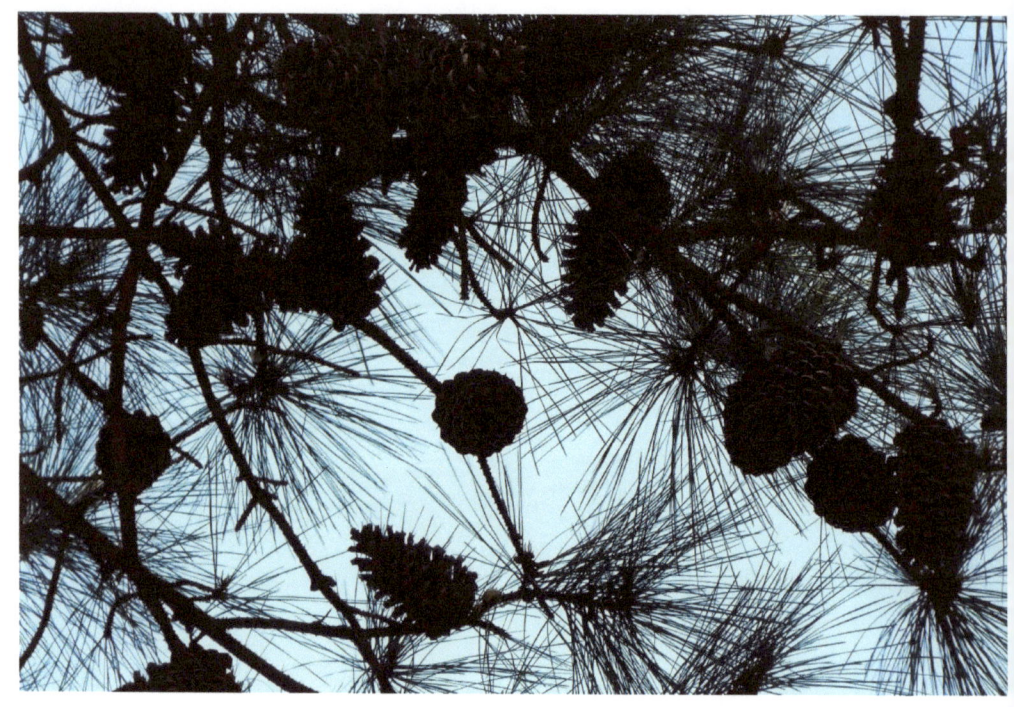

Observe the wonders as they occur around you. Don't claim them.

Feel the artistry moving through, and be silent

 Observa las maravillias que ocurren a tu alrededor. No los reclames.

Siente como se mueve el arte y guarda siliencio

                         Rumi

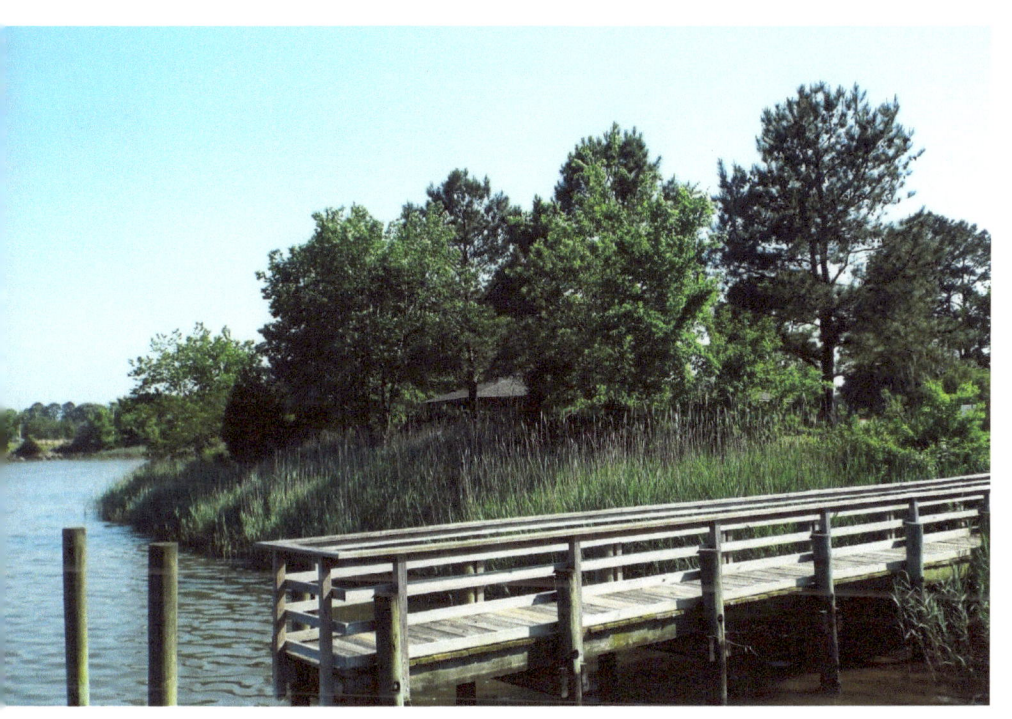

Gone Fishing/ Me Fui a pescar

Saturdays/Sabado

Groceries/Comestibles

Westerns/La pelicula de vacqueros

Today/Hoy dia

Precious one/El mas preciado

Gone fishing/Me Fui a pescar

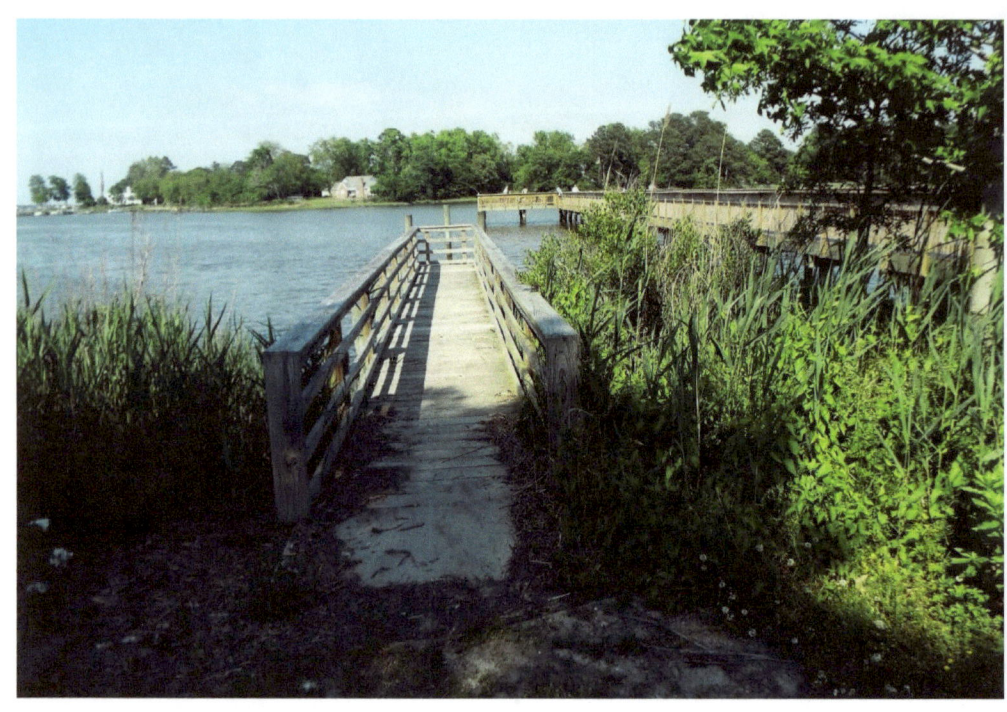

In generosity and helping others be like a river...in modesty and humility be like the earth...in tolerance be like a sea.

En generosidad y ayundando a otros ser como un rio...con modestia y humilidad ser como la tierra…. en tolerancia sea como el mar

                                        Rumi

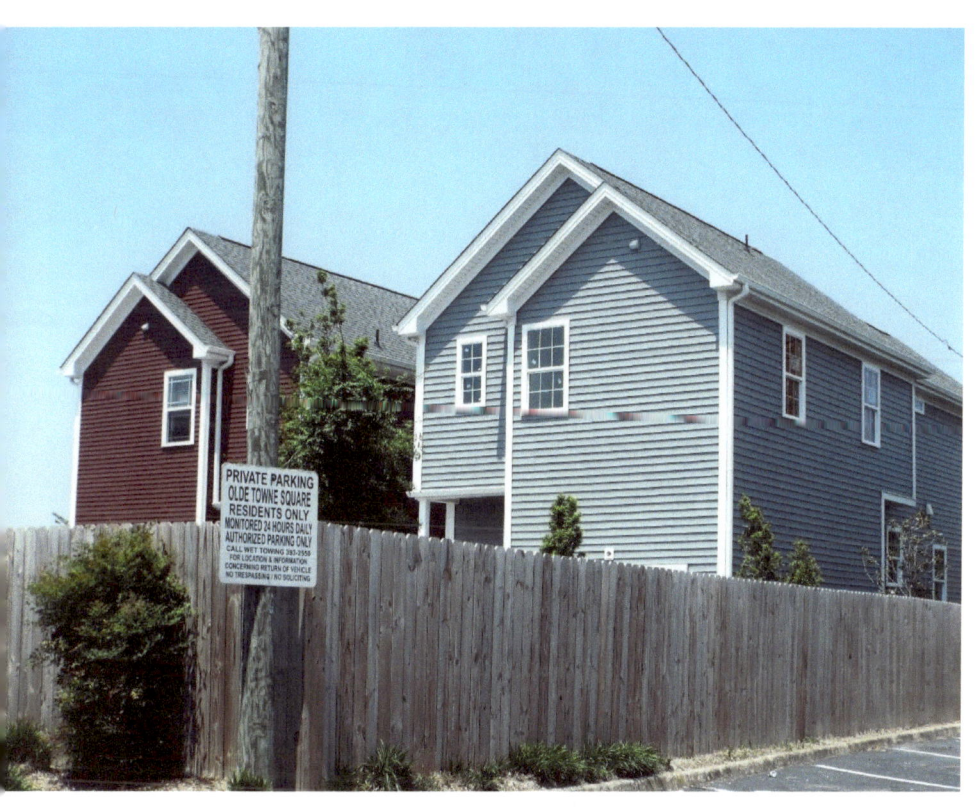

house is made of vinyl and bricks. A Home is a feeling.

na casa esta hecha de vinilo y ladrillos. Un hogar es un sentimiento

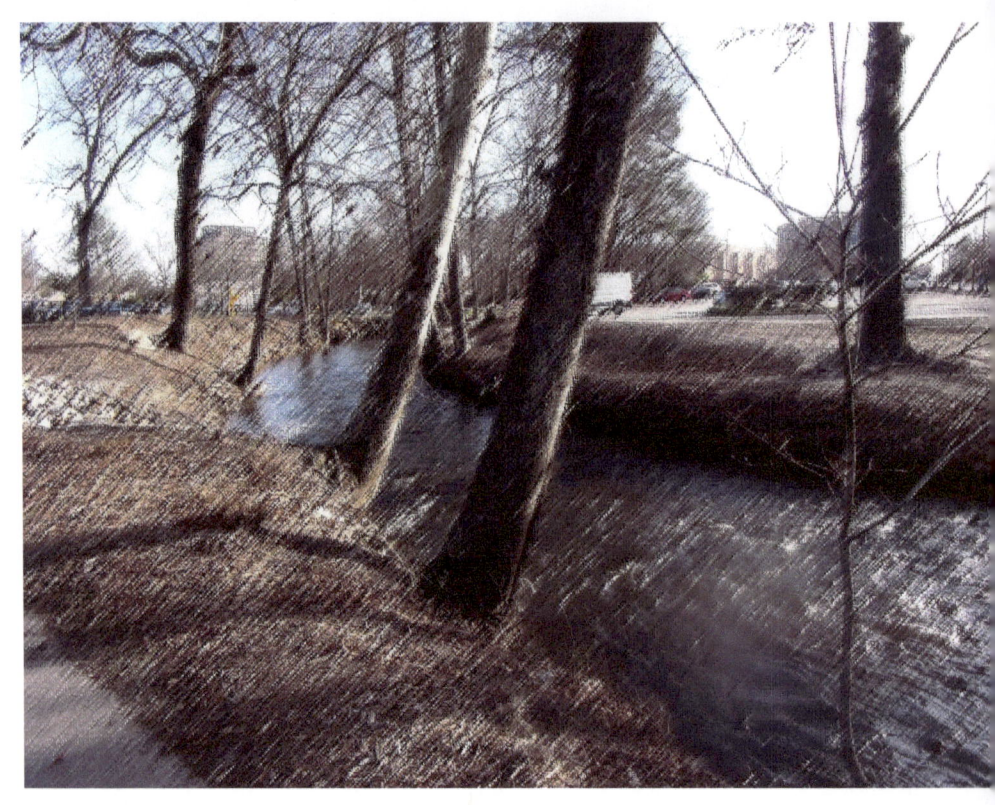

Cape Fear River/Rio del cabo miedo

I am/ Soy

202 blackwater river/202 rios de aquas negras

Central North Carolina/Carolina del norte central

My Source/mi fuente

Haw and Deep River/Haw y rios Profundo

I am flowing/Estoy fluyendo

Downtown Fayetteville, North Carolina/Centro de Fayetteville Carolina del Norte

To/al

Atlantic Ocean/Oceano Atlantico

I am/Soy

Majestic/Majestuoso

I am/Soy

Menacing/Amenazador

Especially/Especialmente

Hurricane/Huracan

Tornado /Tornado

Season/ la Temporada

I leave dead fish/Dojo pescado muerto

On Route 40/en la ruta 40

I am/Soy

Cape Fear/Rio del cabo miedo

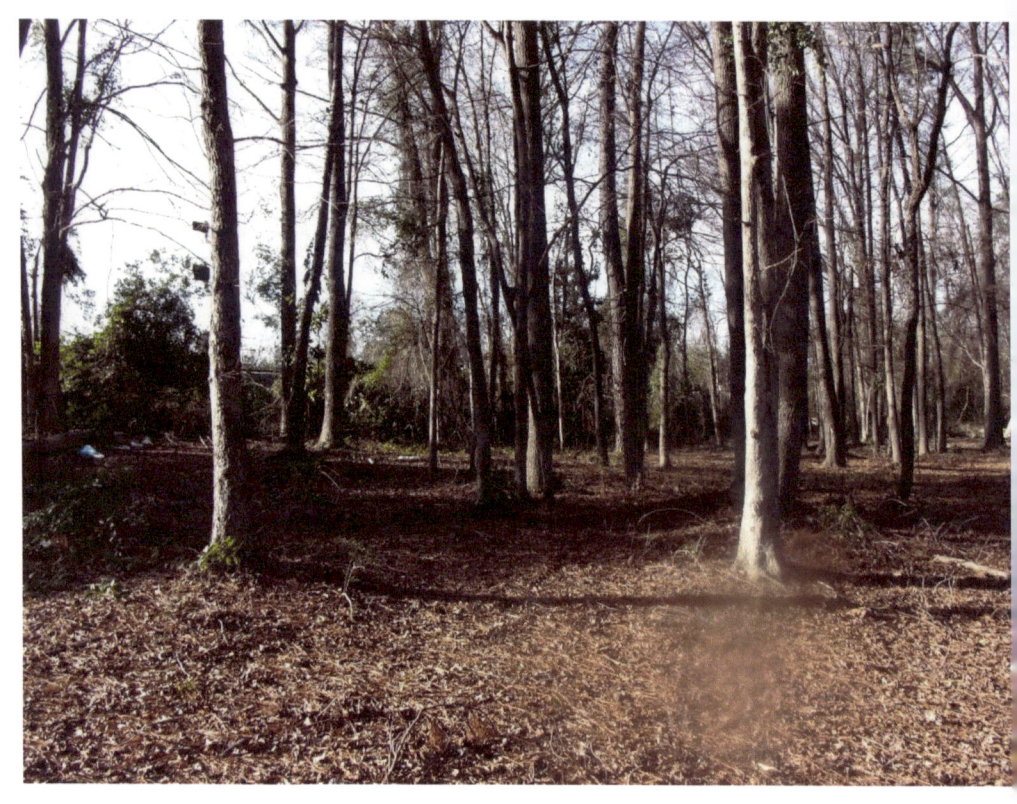

I am whole. I am fulfilled. I have the power to live my life on my terms. I am the final judge of my success.

Estoy complete. Estoy satisfecho. Tengp el poder de vivir mi vida en mis terminos. Soy el juez final de mi exito.

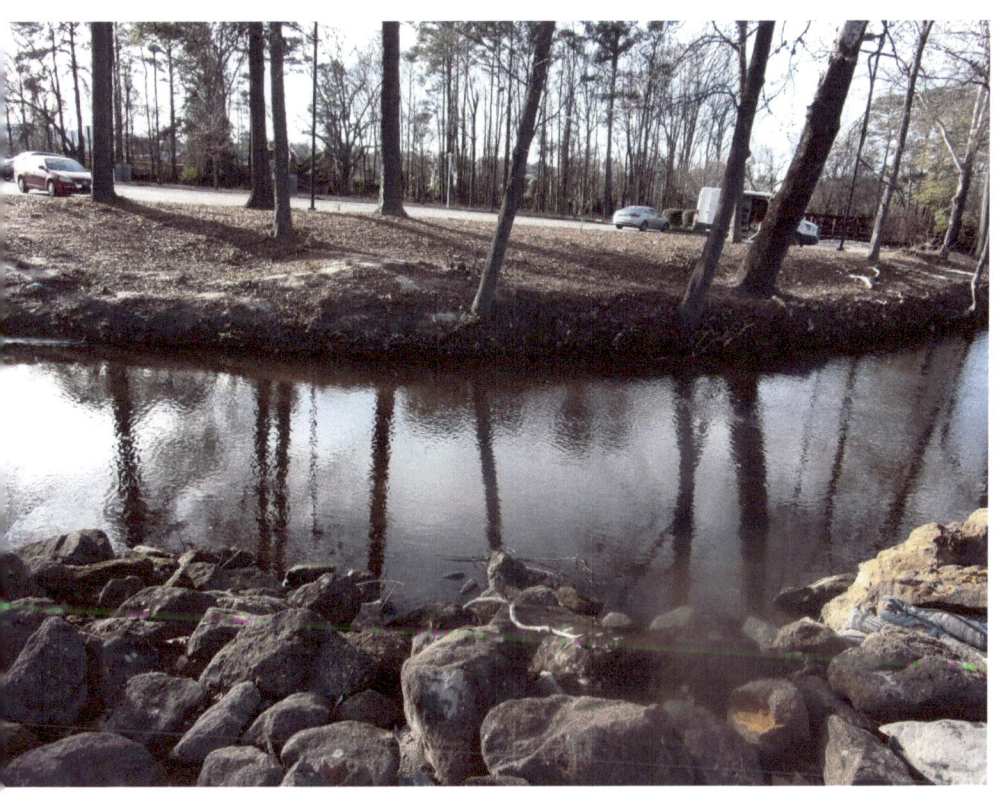

Spirit/Espiritu

You know who you are

You know what you are

You know the voice who is speaking

The voice of power, love, and reason

To sabes quien eres

Sabes lo que eres

Sabes la voz que esta hablando

La voz del poder, el amor y la razon

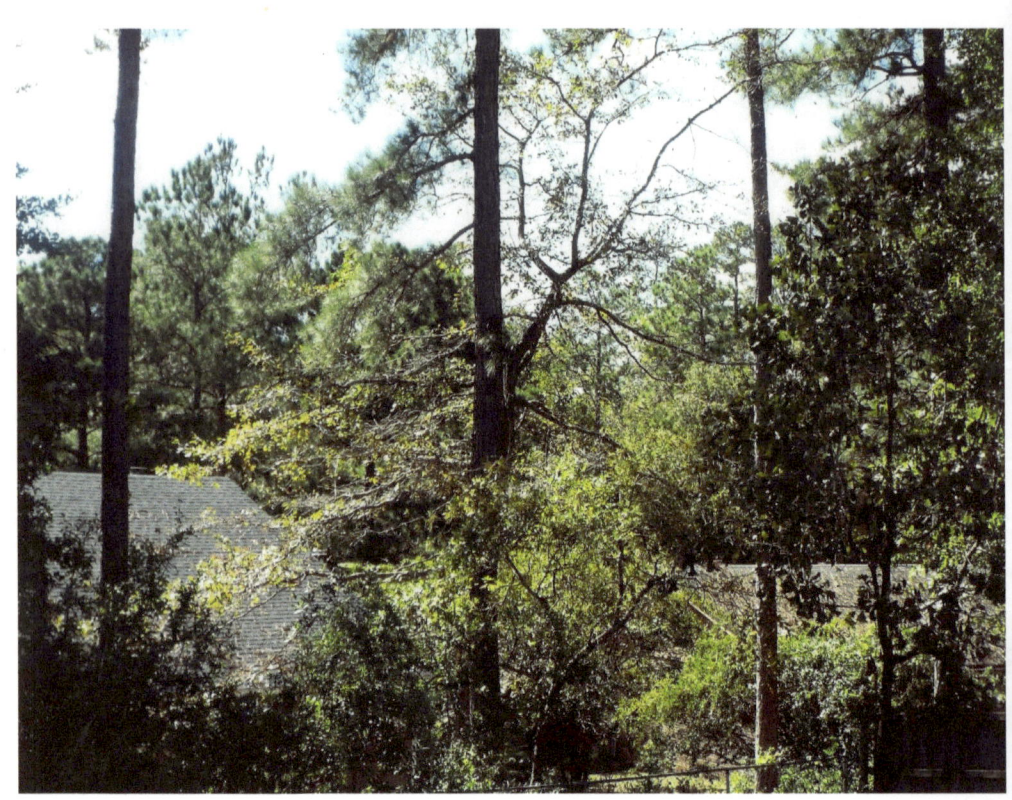

I am whole

I am perfect

I am complete

Estoy completo

Soy perfecto

Estoy complete

Spanish translation of whole and complete are the same word-completo

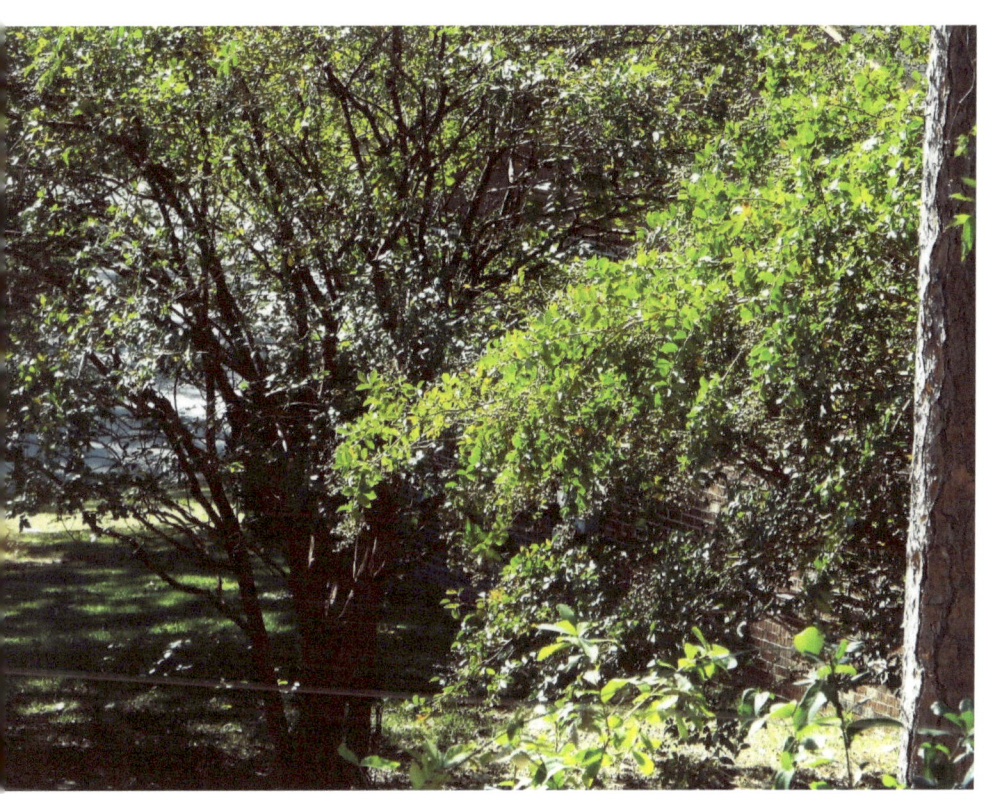

Time/Hora

Time is/Hora es

Today/Hoy

Tomorrow/manana

Yesterday/ayer

Mental concepts/conceptos mentales

Now/Ahora

Reality/Realidad

Eternal/eterno

Cosmos/El Cosmos

Time/Hora

Does not/No

Exist/Existe

Without/sin

Action /El acto

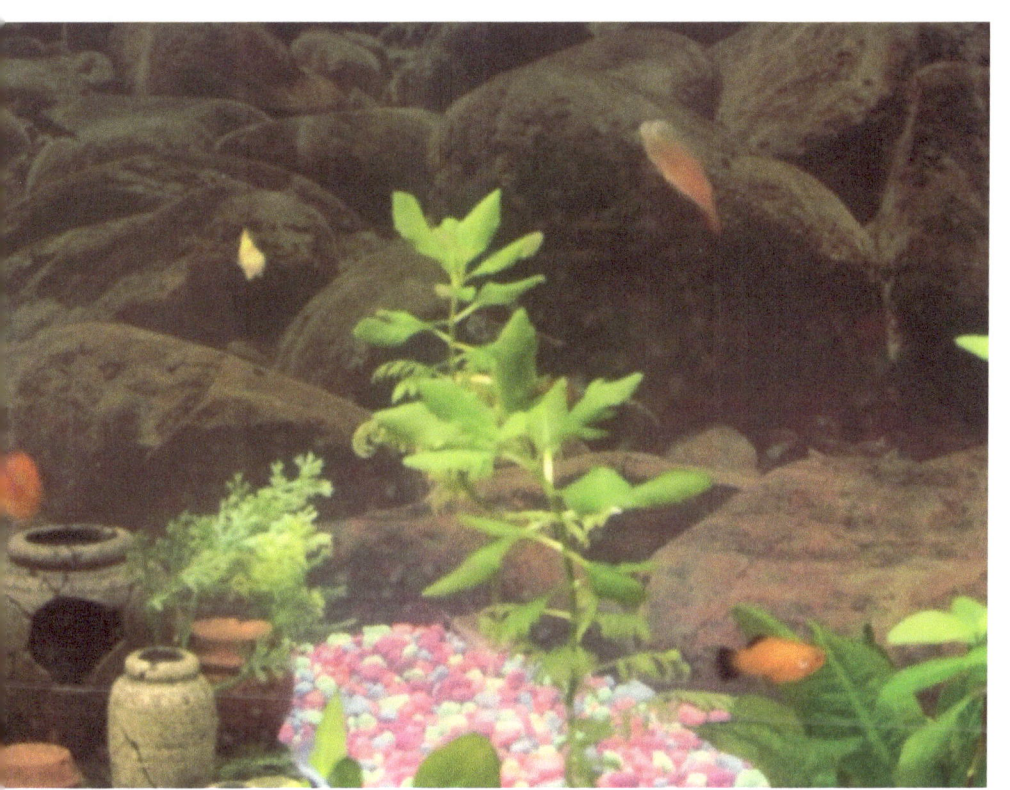

Peaceful/Pacifico

Looking at /Mirando a

Platyfish/Platyfish

Guppies/Guppies

Swordtails/Espadas

Float/flotar

In the water/en el aqua

Dart into/dardo en

Jars/tarros

Behind /detras de

Rocks/las rocas

Lavender candle

Flickering/parpadeo

Darkness/Oscuridad

With only/con solo

Aquarium/La luz de acuario

Light

Peaceful/Pacifico

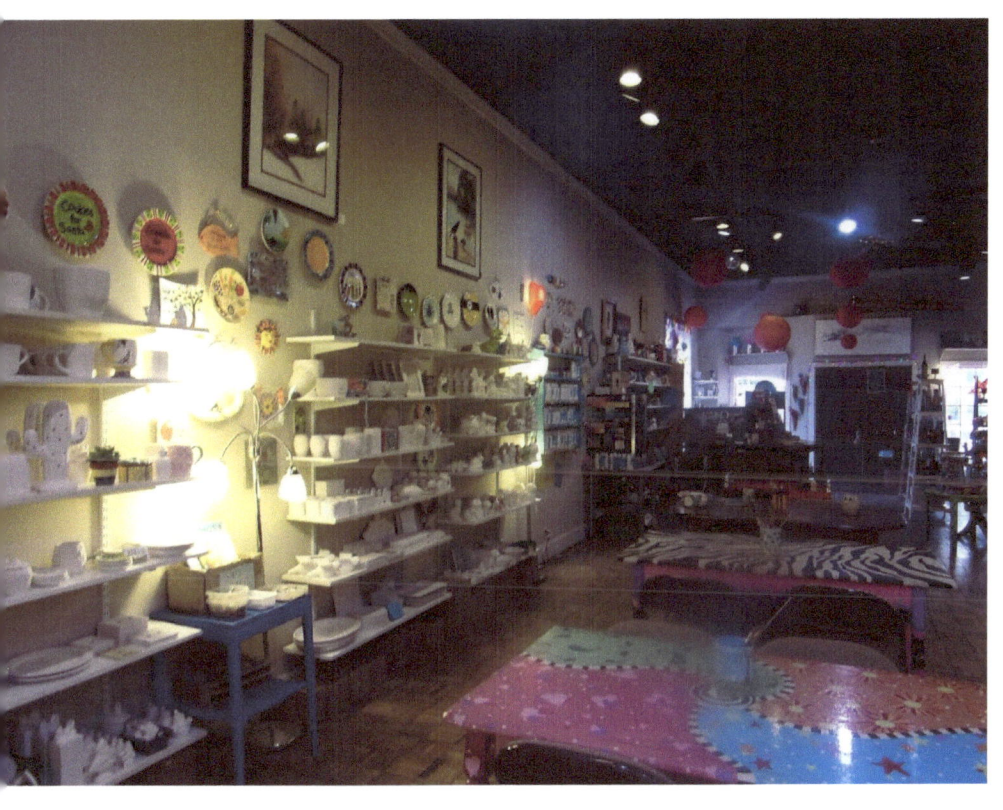

You deserve your own love and affection

Create it

Te mereces tu propio amor y carino

Crearlo

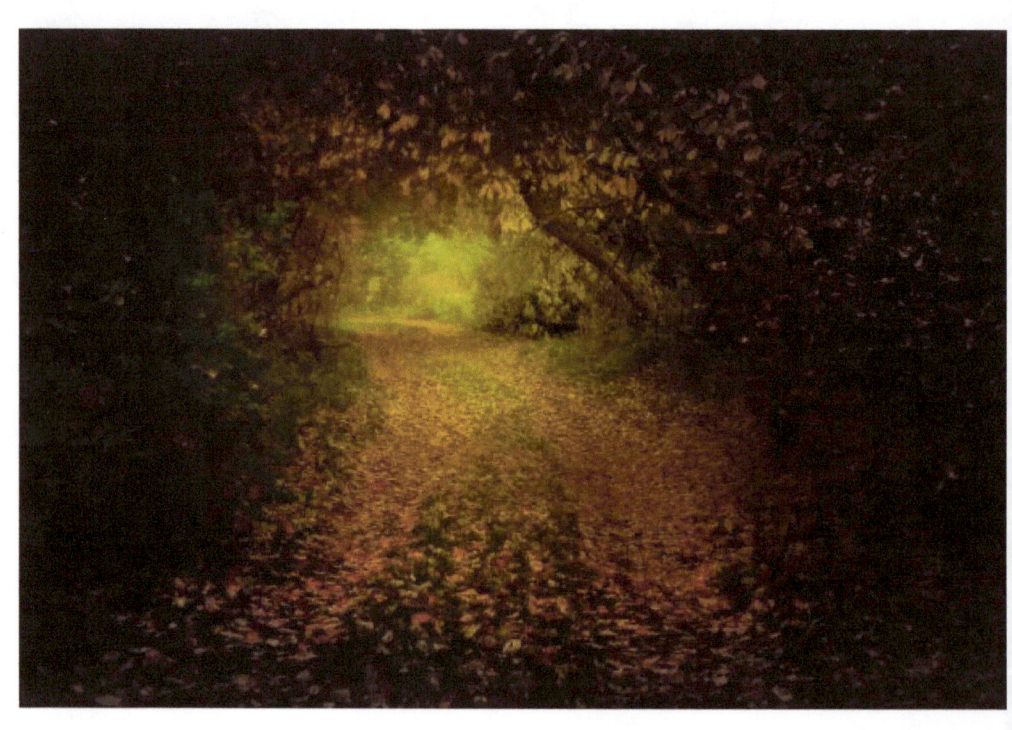

You only lose what you cling to

Solo se pierde lo que afferan a

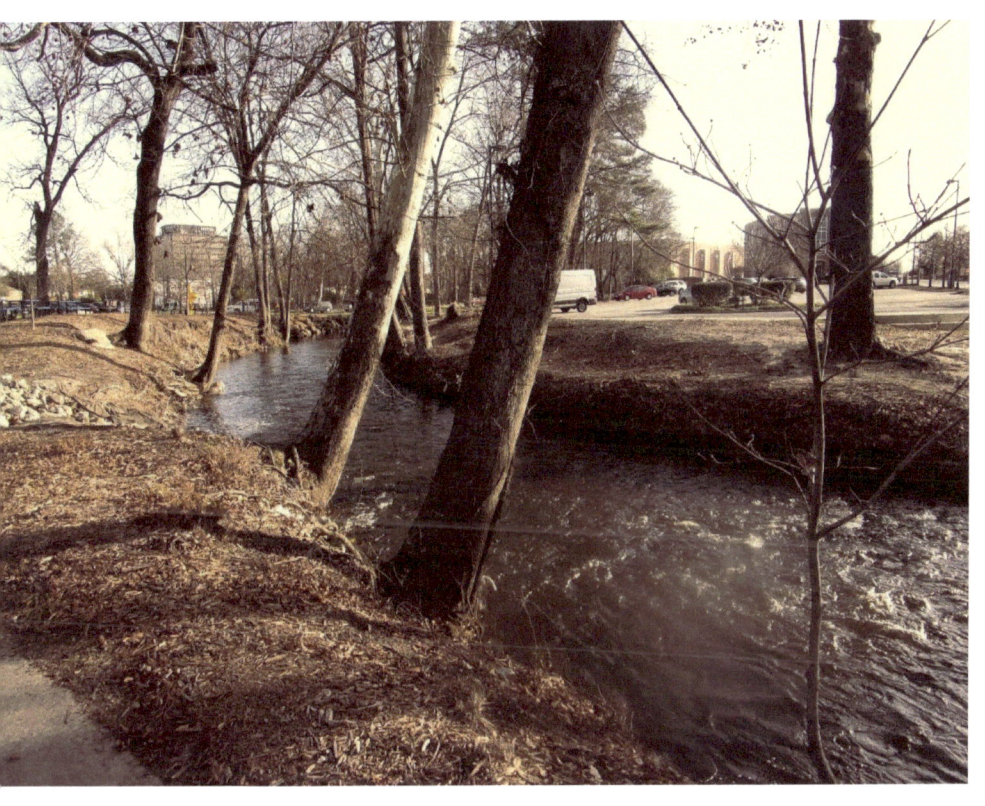

Our thoughts are a moving river

We are shaped by our thoughts

Nuestros pensamientos son un rio en movimiento

Somos formado por nuestro pensamientos.

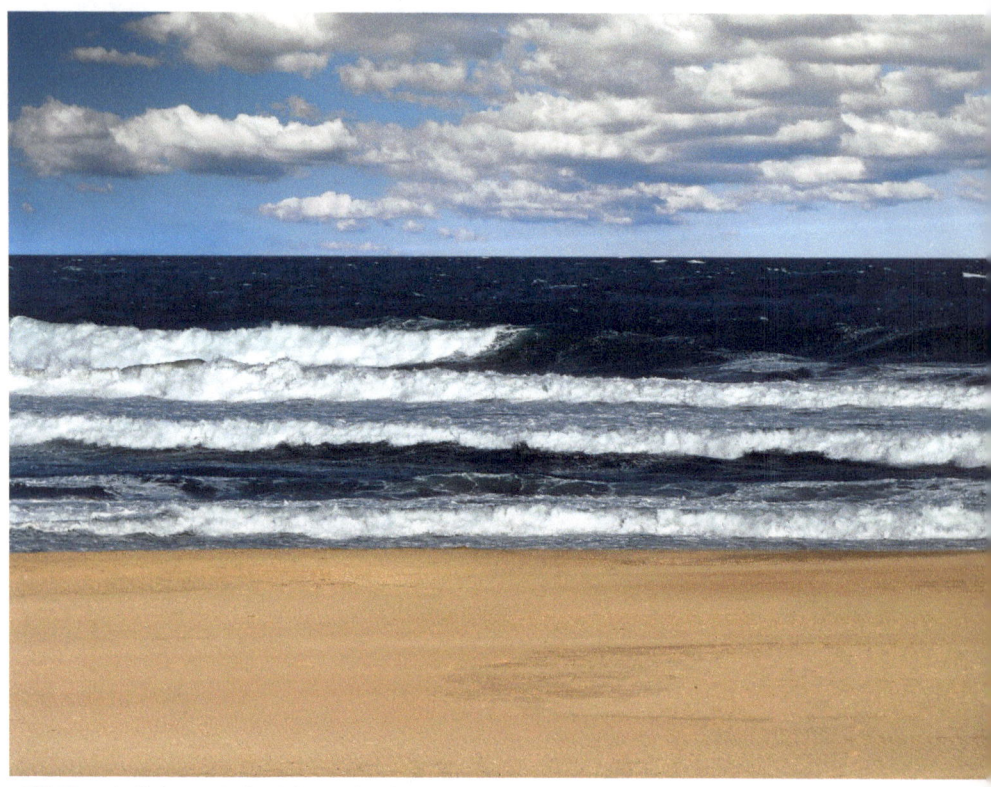

[This Photo](#) by Unknown Author is licensed under [CC BY-SA](#)

Hear the waves within you

Live the roars and whispers

Escucha las olas dentro de ti

Vive los rugidos y susurrus

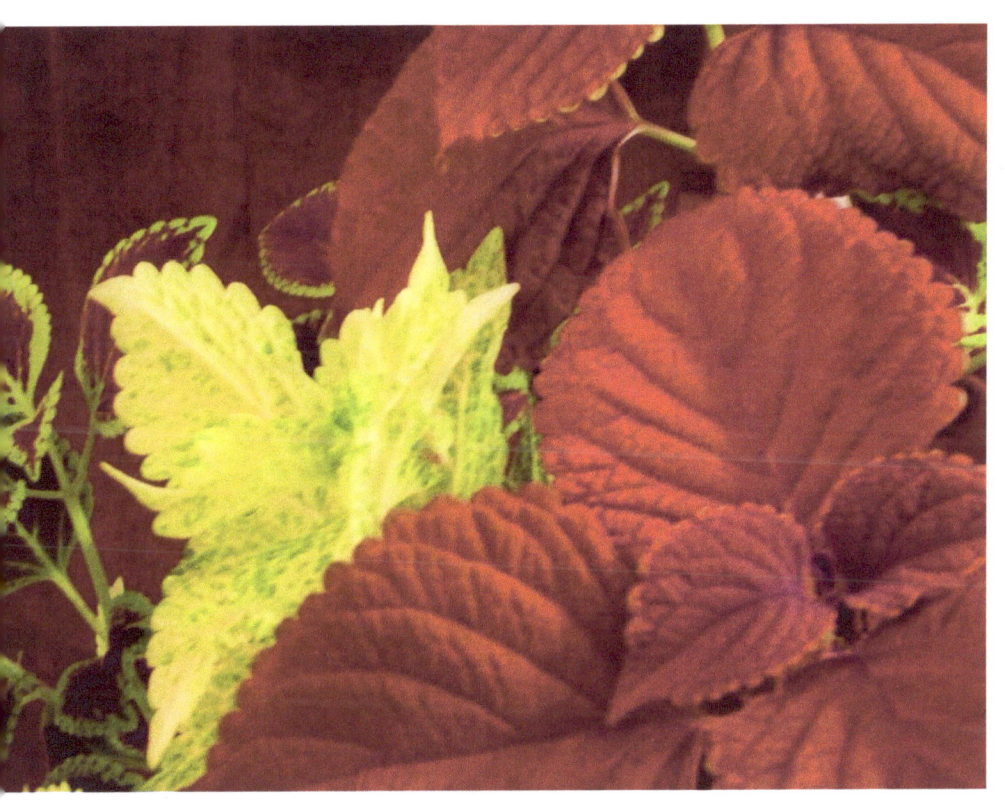

Every experience is a coaching moment

Cada experiencia es un momento de entrenamiento

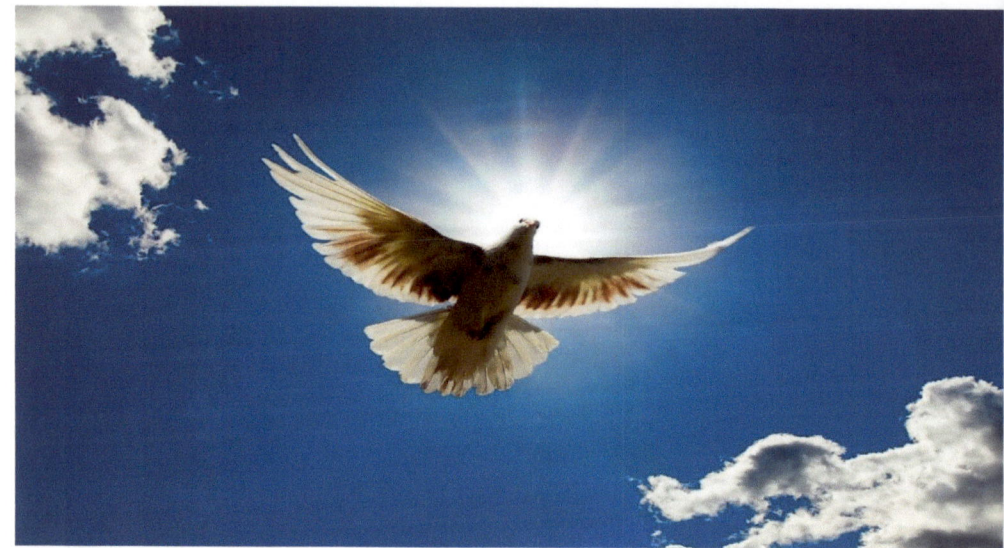

[This Photo](#) by Unknown Author is licensed under [CC BY](#)

I am loving

I am thriving

I am free

To be me

Soy carinosa

Estoy prosperando

Soy libre

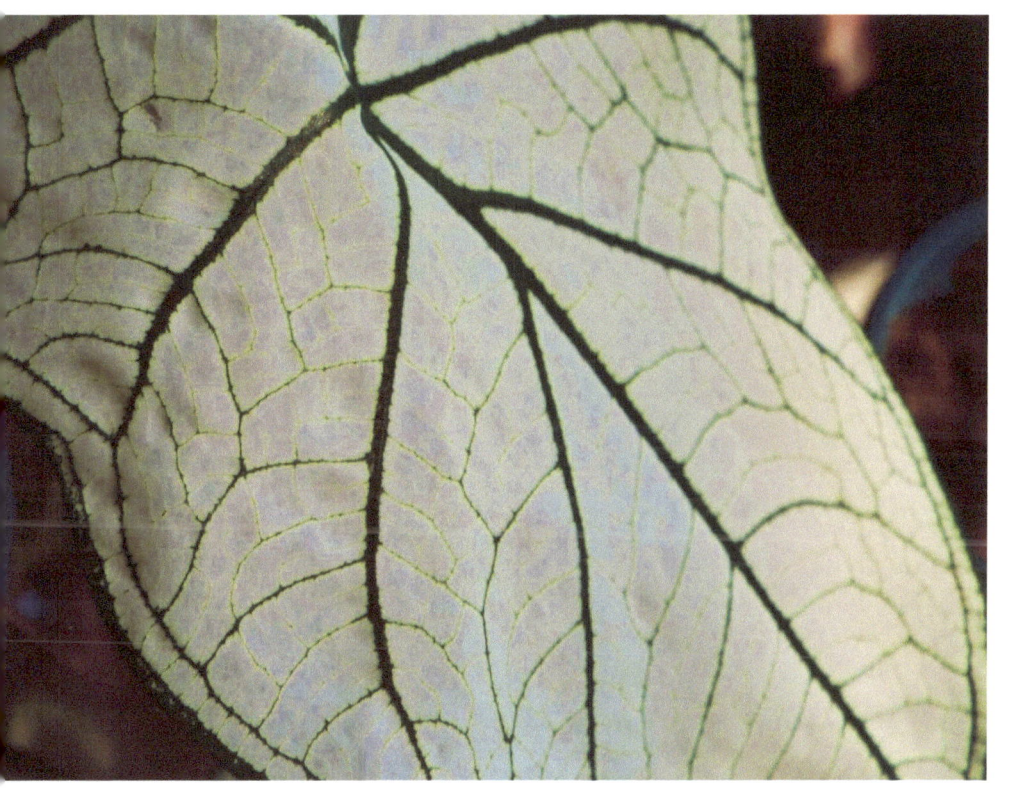

Think only the thoughts you wish to experience

Trust the outcome

Piensa solo los pensamientos que deseas experimentar

Confia en el resultado

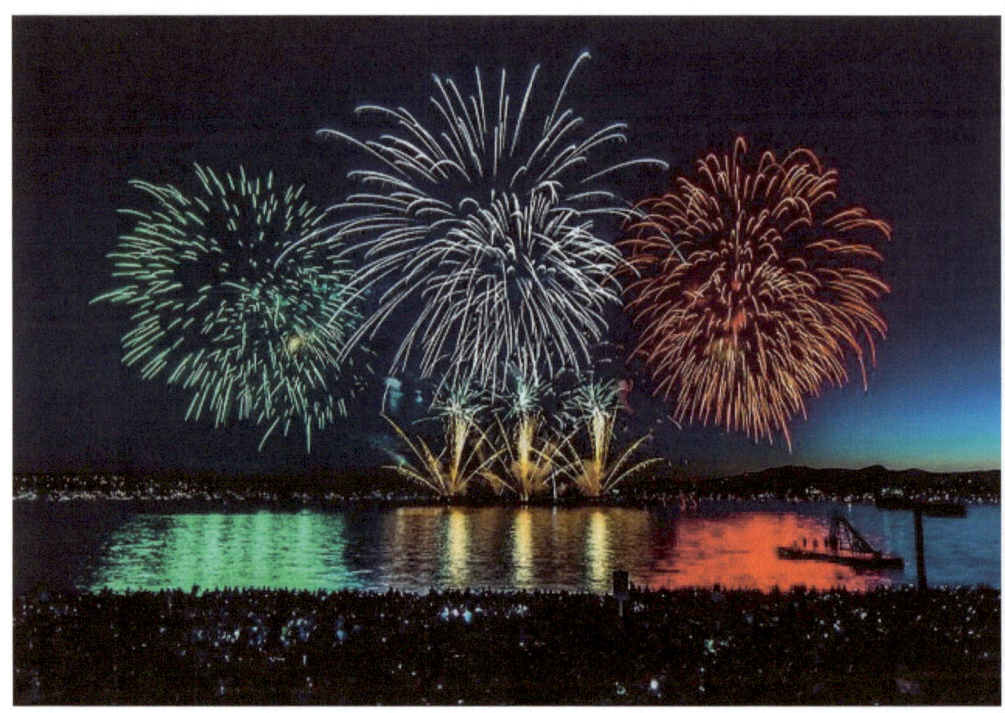

[This Photo](#) by Unknown Author is licensed under CC BY-SA-NC

You have everything you need to live your dream

Tienes todo to que necesitas para vivir tu sueno

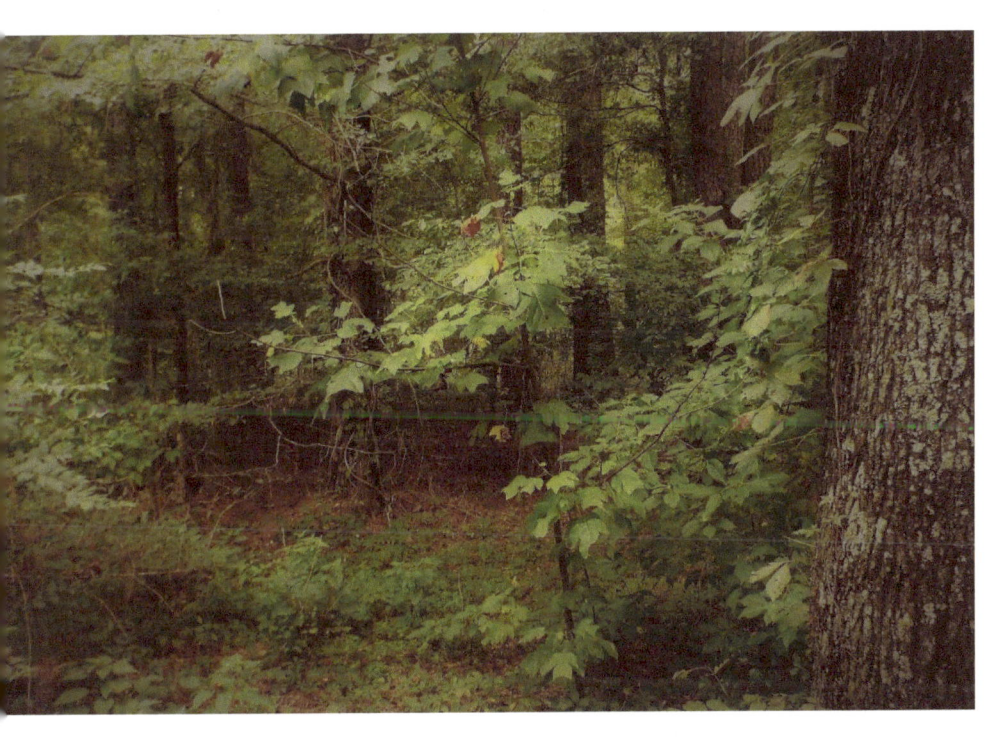

Eden is flourishing in the fullness of identity

Eden esta floreciendo en la plentitude de la indentidad

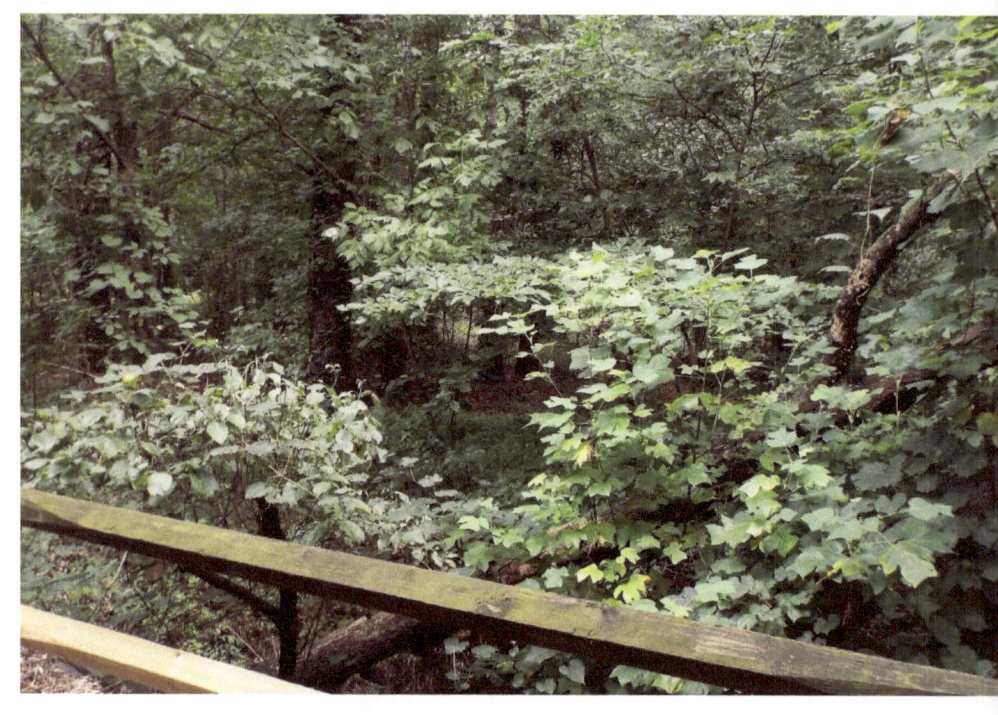

Survival is not taking risks

Living life to the maxium

Putting it all out there

La supervivencia no es tomar riesgos

Viviendo la vida al maximo

Ponlo todo por ahi

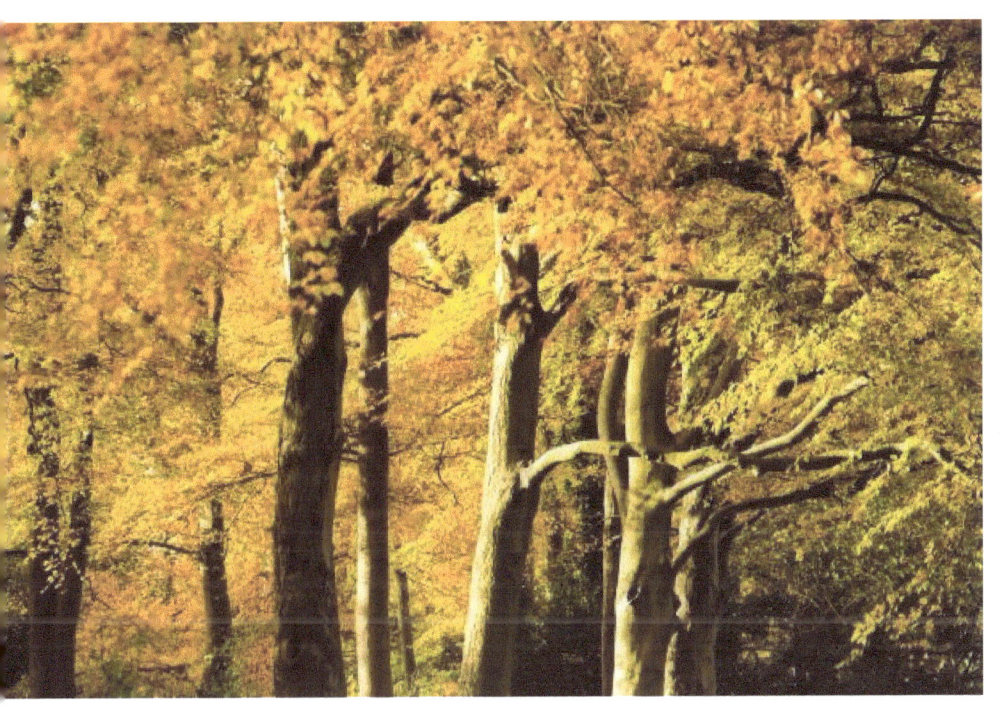

Cost

Our desires can only be fulfilled

At the expense of another

A lie

Costo

Nuestros deseos solo pueden ser cumplidos

A expensas de otros

Una mentira

www.ingramcontent.com/pod-product-compliance
Lightning Source LLC
Chambersburg PA
CBHW041206180526
45172CB00006B/1213